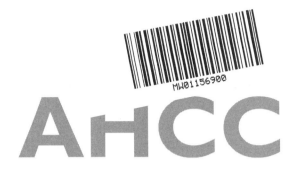

AHCC

The Japanese
Medicinal Mushroom
Immune Enhancer

*Support for Cancer, Chemotherapy Side Effects,
Hepatitis, Inflammation, Fatigue Syndrome,
Viruses & Other Types of Chronic Diseases*

Dan Kenner, LAc.

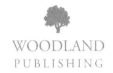

WOODLAND
PUBLISHING

Woodland Publishing
P.O. Box 160
Pleasant Grove, Utah
84062
Visit us at our web site: www.woodlandpublishing.com
or call us toll-free: (800) 777-2665

ISBN 1-58054-340-5
Printed in the United States of America

Contents

Introduction

PEOPLE ARE NATURALLY skeptical when someone makes extravagant claims for healing methods or healing substances. The dominant approach in health care in our culture is based on the notion of specific diseases and specific medications for specific diseases. It evokes surprise when a popular medicine like aspirin, well known for the treatment of pain, is found to have other properties; i.e., the ability to thin the blood to protect the heart. With today's abundance of new nutritional supplements and the accompanying promotional literature glowing with enthusiastic claims, separating the wheat from the chaff has become more difficult.

In the case of AHCC, a "superfood" nutritional supplement from Japan, there is an unusual combination of mainstream acceptance by the medical profession and by the general public. In fact, AHCC is close to being considered a mainstream cancer therapy in Japan, and its acceptance is rapidly growing in other countries. Part of this rapid acceptance is due to the volume of scientific research devoted to the many applications of AHCC. AHCC is being used in over 700 hospitals in Japan and is being researched in fifteen Japanese medical colleges and universities. Outside of Japan, universities in United States, China, Korea and Thailand are conducting research on AHCC.

Health care professionals advocate the use of AHCC for the treatment of cancer, AIDS, hepatitis C, diabetes, hypertension, autoimmune diseases and many other afflictions. This wide range of applications is causing many physicians and researchers to adopt a different viewpoint about many chronic and life-threatening diseases. Perhaps lung cancer is not a disease of the lung, and perhaps hepatitis is not a disease of the liver. Perhaps these are both diseases of the immune system. A failure or deterioration of key immune functions could be the factor that links numerous health disorders of aging or degeneration together, even though we've studied them as separate diseases in the past.

From this emerging point of view on the nature and origin of disease, one could say that the white blood cells of the immune system need AHCC the way the blood needs iron, the bones need calcium or the nerves need phosphorus. This direct nourishment of the white blood cells is one reason we can consider AHCC a superfood. Another reason is because it is extremely absorbable and digestible due to its low molecular weight. There is no reason to doubt that AHCC is one nutritional supplement that has universal application not only for treatment of disease, but also for maintenance of optimum health.

Healing Traditions

A pickling crock was once an important feature of a traditional Japanese kitchen. The pickling crock was a way to preserve vegetables without refrigeration. Fresh vegetables were placed in a combination of rice bran and sea salt for days and even weeks, just as German housewives preserved cabbage for the winter as sauerkraut. Not only does the pickling process preserve vegetables harvested during the warm months for winter consumption, but the fermentation enhances their nutritional value. The salt fermentation results in the growth of friendly microbes and enzymes improving digestibility and efficiency as a food.

Not only did the Japanese traditionally preserve vegetables for food, but they also prepared medicines using these processes. The shiitake mushroom is a medicinal mushroom used for food. Rare and precious mushrooms such as the reishi mushroom were cherished for their medicinal properties. Preserving these mushrooms to maintain health and longevity are part of the Japanese tradition of healing. Even today after modernization, the Japanese are noted for their longevity. The Japanese are possibly the largest per capita consumers of herbs and nutritional supplements in the world. Out of all of the herbs and supplements available in Japan there is one that stands out as the most well-researched, powerful and sought-after supplements is the superfood known as AHCC.

What is AHCC?

AHCC is a mildly sweet tasting monosaccharide produced from the mycelium of a shiitake hybrid grown in rice bran extract. Rice bran itself is known to have antiviral and immune-system-supporting effects. AHCC was developed in 1987 at the University of Tokyo Faculty of Pharmaceutical Sciences by Dr. Toshihiko Okamoto in a joint effort with researchers of the Amino Up Chemical Co., Ltd.

AHCC is extracted from the mycelial threads of the mushroom blend, which are grown in a pre-cultivation tank. The mushroom colonies are further cultured in the main cultivation tank for forty-five days. AHCC is obtained in a patented process of cultivation, enzymatic decomposition, sterilization, concentration and freeze-drying. Among other important components, AHCC contains partially acetylated a-glucan, which is known to have beneficial effects on the immune system.

One advantage of the fermentation process is that it breaks down nutrients into a more absorbable form that is easily integrated into the system. AHCC has a molecular weight of only 5,000 daltons. The molecular weight of most mushroom extracts is in the hundreds of thousands of daltons. This low molecular weight increases the efficiency of the nutrients such that all available nutrients are absorbed and used, rather than eliminated. This small molecular weight also means that the potent nutrients in AHCC can be assimilated quickly by the white blood cells for immediate use in destruction of tumors or strengthening of the body's defenses. This, along with its immune-strengthening functions, is another reason why AHCC can be called a superfood.

The letters AHCC stand for active hexose correlated compound. It was originally developed in the late 1980s to be a natural agent for regulating high blood pressure. Researchers soon observed its many beneficial effects on the immune system. AHCC has been used to treat some of mankind's most grave afflictions including cancer, heart disease, hepatitis and AIDS. AHCC has been widely publicized in Japan in literally hundreds of newspaper and magazine articles, as well as in peer review scientific journals. AHCC is the subject of several books in Japan such as *Testimony of 11 Cancer Doctors: Why Is AHCC Effective?* Gendai Shorin, Tokyo 1999; *The Cancer Immunity Screening*, K.Uno, Metamor shuppan, Tokyo 2000.

In addition, there have been anecdotal claims of cure of or improvement of numerous other afflictions including slow wound healing, stomach ulcers, gum disease, fatigue syndrome, parasites, multiple sclerosis and other autoimmune diseases.

Why is AHCC So Versatile?

How is it possible that one substance can be effective in treating so many health problems? The answer is twofold. Part of the answer lies in the fact that AHCC goes beyond being a medication for treating disease. As a "superfood," it nourishes the body at a very fundamental level—the body's immunity. The other part of the answer is in our perception of disease. When we define *disease*, we often look at the system of the body where the symptoms arise and the type of lesion in that system. For example, if there is a circulation problem we look at the heart or arteries and look for a specific type of damage. If there is lung cancer, we treat the lung. If it's prostate cancer, then we treat the prostate gland. In hepatitis we aim at treatment of the liver, and so forth. Only recently has medical science begun to explore the idea that some health problems are diseases of the whole system, not just one of the parts. The immune system is a good index of the health of the whole body because its activity spans all of the other systems of the body. The immune system's activity intimately affects each organ and system at a fundamental level.

Oncologist and cancer researcher Katsuaki Uno, M.D., a proponent of the use of AHCC for cancer treatment says:

> Individual cancer cells certainly arise from genetic abnormalities. However, for cancer cells to grow into a tumor requires the development of a "diseased condition" resulting from the decline of immune strength. In other words, cancer is an abnormality of immunity that brings about the onset of disease—it's a disease of immunity. This viewpoint implies a compelling notion. These days many specialists have come to realize that abnormalities of immunity play a fundamental role in the deterioration of "diseases of lifestyle," conditions in which the system is overtaxed, such as arteriosclerosis and high blood pressure, into the onset of cerebral vascular disease, cardiovascular disease, diabetes and other conditions.

Dr. Uno explains that the ability of the immune system to dispose of abnormal cells can become impaired so the abnormal cells, cancer cells or others, can accumulate in the tissues. The AIDS problem forced scientists to take a closer look at the workings of the immune system. AIDS was the first disease specifically identified as a disease of immunity. It is now known that HIV infection alone does not cause AIDS. If the immune system is weakened, it then becomes possible for the HIV to take hold and do its damage to the whole body.

The Importance of Immunity to Infection

Besides preventing cancer and AIDS, another important function of the immune system is to protect the body from microbes that cause infections. Recently scientists have discovered a possible microbe connection in many chronic diseases that were previously not considered to be infections. A microbe connection has been identified in such diseases as arteriosclerosis, heart disease, Alzheimer's disease, duodenal ulcers, diabetes, SLE (systemic lupus erythematosus), rheumatoid arthritis, Hashimoto's thyroiditis, multiple sclerosis, most forms of cancer, polycystic ovary disease, some

---

CLINICAL AND LABORATORY EVIDENCE FOR EFFICACY OF AHCC

AHCC has been used successfully to treat the following health conditions:

- Cancer: liver, breast, prostate, gastrointestinal, multiple myeloma
- Precancerous conditions: cervical dysplasia
- Human Immunovirus (HIV)
- Hepatitis C and cirrhosis of the liver
- Chronic infections
- Diabetes
- Stress
- High blood pressure, cardiac arrhythmia
- Glaucoma

types of inflammatory bowel disease, cerebral palsy and even most major psychiatric diseases. The list doesn't end there.

There are many other conditions that could possibly be caused by microbes: including obesity and eating disorders, and a number of diseases with less-familiar names. As support for this new "germ theory" grows, the implication that the ability of the immune system to control these disease-causing microbes could be a major factor in the onset and progression of these diseases. It is known that in hospitals, doctors, nurses and administrative personnel all test positive for microbes like staphylococcus, but only the people with compromised immunity (the patients) actually come down with infections. The immune system, which spans the boundaries of all of the body's vital systems, could be the key factor in understanding the cause of chronic and degenerative disease. Let's take a look at this important system that protects the integrity of all the other vital systems of the body.

Guided Tour of the Immune System

The immune system is found throughout the body. Much of it is located in the lymphatic system, which circulates the tissue fluid that bathes all of the body's cells in nutrients and chemical messengers. The tissue fluid also carries away the waste products of metabolism from the cells. The immune system is also made up of many types of cells. The spleen, the tonsils, the adenoids, the thymus gland and the Peyer's patches in the small intestine are all lymphoid tissue. The mucous membranes and bone marrow also play important roles in immunity.

Lymphocytes and White Blood Cells

Lymphocytes are white blood cells formed in lymphoid tissue. There are different kinds of lymphocytes and other white blood cells in the immune system that have different functions. They may destroy foreign proteins or invading microbes or produce chemicals that act as messengers that stimulate or suppress other immune cells. Some of the chemicals act as a type of memory, so the body can recognize an infectious agent it has previously encountered in order to respond more rapidly and effectively.

IMMUNE SYSTEM COMPONENTS THAT PROTECT THE CELLS FROM CANCER AND CHRONIC DISEASE

WHITE BLOOD CELLS:

- *macrophages*– "eat up" abnormal cells and invaders

- *natural killer cells (NK)*– "explode" abnormal cells and invaders

- *lymphokine activated killer cells (LAK)*– another type of killer cell

- *neutrophils*– white blood cell similar to a macrophage

- *cytotoxic lymphocytes (killer T cells)*– destroy invading organisms and abnormal cells (malignant or virus-infected)

CYTOKINES (Chemical Messengers Between Cells)

- *interferon (gamma interferon)*– protects cells from viruses, destroys cancer tumors and stimulates NK activity

- *interleukin-2 (IL-2)*– stimulates growth and activity of T cells

- *interleukin-12 (IL-12)*– stimulates NK cells and strengthens cellular immunity

- *tumor necrosis factor (TNF)*– induces tumor destruction

Most of the active components of the immune system are white blood cells, also called leukocytes. There are several different types and subtypes of white blood cells. There are several that are important to immune protection. Macrophages (literally "big eater" in Greek) are developed from cells called monocytes that are formed in the bone marrow. Macrophages ingest bacteria and other substances in a process called "phagocytosis" (literally means "cell eating"). Phagocytosis is mainly carried out by the macrophages and white blood cells called neutrophils.

The Immune Response

The immune response depends on its ability to recognize a foreign protein or other particle as abnormal. Abnormal foreign particles are called "antigens." Macrophages circulate throughout the body and consume any antigens they encounter, then carry them to lymph nodes to white cells called helper T cells. T cells, or T lymphocytes, are involved in various specific immune responses. There are many different subtypes including helper T cells, suppressor T cells, cytotoxic T cells, and delayed hypersensitivity T cells.

One important group of lymphocytes is the specialized group of cells called natural killer (NK) cells. Natural killer cells, as well as macrophages, can destroy tumor cells as well as microbes. Both NK cells and macrophages appear to play a role in immune surveillance. Immune surveillance is a protective mechanism by which abnormal cells are detected and destroyed on first exposure before they multiply and create a clinical problem. This function of immune surveillance is possibly the most critical function to protect the body from chronic and degenerative diseases. Macrophages engulf and digest the particles they destroy but NK cells use a different mechanism. NK cells, like heat-seeking missiles, attach themselves to the surface of microbe, cancer cells or other substances and inject a "granule" into the interior of its "prey." The granule causes a chemical reaction that makes the cancer cell or bacteria "explode," often within only a few minutes.

Cytokines—Intercellular Messengers

Cytokines are chemical messengers that communicate between cells to direct and to enhance immune response. One of the best known is interferon, a family of proteins that inhibit the spread of viruses. When a virus invades a cell, the cells immune mechanism releases interferon, which binds to other cells and triggers the synthesis of protective substances within these cells that prevent viral invasion. All cells manufacture interferon if they are stimulated in the right way. Interferon also probably plays a role in protecting the body from cancer. Some cancers are thought to be caused by viruses, but interferon also seems to help with tumors that are not caused by viruses. Interferon also stimulates and enhances the activity of both macrophages and natural killer (NK) cells.

SUMMARY OF THE EFFECTS OF AHCC ON THE IMMUNE SYSTEM

- Increases the number of T cells as much as 200 percent
- Activates the immune cells involved in "surveillance": NK cells, LAK cells and macrophages
- Increases production of cytokines: TNF-a, gamma-interferon, IL-2 and IL-12
- Inhibits immunosuppressive cytokines like TGF-b
- Improves Th1/Th2 balance (cellular vs. humoral immunity)

Other important cytokines are interleukin-2 (IL-2) and interleukin-12 (IL-12). IL-2 is also known as "T cell growth factor." IL-12 also activates suppressor T cells and also natural killer (NK) cells. When stimulated by IL-12, NK cells begin to produce gamma interferon, an especially powerful immune agent. Another important biologically active group of proteins called "tumor necrosis factor" (TNF) may also have cytokine functions. TNF helps to induce a fever response and to destroy cancer cells by inducing cell death (known scientifically as "apoptosis").

Natural Killer (NK) Cell Activity

When activated, these cells are extremely dynamic eliminators of foreign matter. They comprise about 15 percent of the body's white blood cells. There are seldom too few NK cells in the system; what is important is how active they are. Their ability to recognize and destroy invading or abnormal cells depends on their mobility and the number of granules they contain. These "explosive" granules are injected into the foreign or abnormal cell causing it to break apart. The most important fact about NK cells is that they selectively destroy abnormal cells and foreign microbes.

The activity of NK cells is one of the best ways to evaluate the prognosis of a patient with cancer or AIDS. The lower the activity of the NK cells, the shorter the likely time of survival. When NK cell activity stops, it is a sign of imminent death. The activity of NK cells can be measured by a test called the NK cell function test, also known as the four-hour chromium-release assay. The test is straightforward. The patient's blood is placed in a container holding live cancer cells and the percentage of cancer cells destroyed by the patient's blood is measured after four hours. The more active the NK cells in the blood are, the higher the measured percentage will be. It is necessary to test for NK cell cytotoxic activity to know the capability of the immune system in cancer and chronic disease. This test is becoming more common and is now available in many conventional labs. Low NK cell activity has also been associated with fatigue, chronic viral infections, autoimmune diseases and malignant tumors.

Research has shown that AHCC increases NK cell activity by increasing the number of explosive granules they contain. The use of AHCC has increased the activity of NK cells by 300 percent and even gradually increasing to as high as 800 percent over time.

Effects of AHCC on Cytokines

AHCC induces the production of the cytokines that stimulate cellular immunity. It increases the number of T lymphocytes by up to 200 percent. There is also evidence that AHCC increases the population of macrophages, even doubling them. AHCC also inhibits an immune suppressive factor that promotes tumor growth.

AHCC Supports Immunity—Even in Cancer Chemotherapy

The effects of the assault to the immune system from cytotoxic chemotherapy for cancer are well known. The suppression of the immune system makes the patient extremely susceptible to infections. Low immunity can also create conditions for cancer cells to proliferate. One study at Hokkaido University in Japan showed that AHCC can reverse the suppression of immunity caused by chemotherapy by increasing macrophage activity and increase IL-12 levels, although there may be additional mechanisms.

Treating Chronic and Life-Threatening Diseases with AHCC

Cancer

Cancer is possibly the most feared word in the English language. The accepted conventional methods of treatment are chemotherapy, radiation and surgery. All of these approaches radically affect the patient's immunity and well-being. Chemotherapy and radiation not only weaken immunity, but chemotherapy in particular damages the patient's well-being by causing loss of appetite, nausea, vomiting, depression, fatigue and loss of hair. Chemotherapy often adversely affects liver function, which can cause numerous complications.

In addition, there is often damage to the bone marrow, injuring the immune system at a deep level and affecting the body's ability to produce red and white blood cells. The newest trend in cancer therapy is for nontoxic treatment to boost the immune system. This immunotherapy uses "biological response modifiers" (BRM) and is rapidly gaining credibility even in conventional medical circles, especially in Japan where AHCC often accompanies mainstream cancer treatment. In Japan, AHCC is widely considered to be the strongest known immune system strengthening biological response modifier.

What types of cancer are indicated? Because AHCC is a medical "superfood" that strengthens immune system function, it could be recommended for any type of cancer. Data from the treatment of over 100,000 cancer patients with various types of cancer has shown that 60 percent of patients have benefitted to some degree and many have found it effective enough to induce remission.

AHCC has shown itself to be particularly effective for liver, lung, stomach, colon, breast, thyroid, ovarian, testicular, tongue, kidney and pancreatic cancers. Results range from actual reduction of tumor mass, arresting tumor growth, stopping the spread of the tumor throughout the body (metastasis), increased survival time, and very significantly, improvement of the quality of life.

SUMMARY OF EFFICACY OF AHCC IN CANCER TREATMENT

- AHCC has been effective in 60 percent of cancer patients
- AHCC reduces tumor size often shrinking them completely
- AHCC can inhibit metastasis and recurrence of cancer
- Increases patients' survival periods
- Improves patients' conditions with no side effects
- Mitigates or eliminates the side effects of chemotherapy
- Restores NK cell activity suppressed by chemotherapy
- Combined with chemotherapy, reduced primary tumors by 20% more than chemotherapy alone
- Particularly effective for cancers of the liver, stomach, colon, breast, thyroid ovaries, testicles, tongue, kidneys and pancreas

Improves survival rate: In one landmark study in Osaka, Japan, AHCC was given to liver cancer patients following surgery. In comparison to a control group who received no AHCC, the rate of survival after five years was 14 percent higher in the AHCC group. By the time the study had ended, 79 percent of the group taking AHCC was alive compared to 51 percent of the control group. In addition, the post-operative occurrence of hepatitis and cirrhosis was reduced according to laboratory test evidence measured even as much as five years later. More significantly, fewer patients had recurrence of cancer: 49 percent in the AHCC group compared to 67 percent in the control group. The survival rate among the participants who took AHCC was an average of twenty-three months longer.

AHCC for the side effects of cancer treatment. The authors of the liver cancer study noted that there were no undesirable side effects reported in the group who took AHCC. This is what we would expect from a nutrient, but beyond the fact that there were no unpleasant side effects from AHCC, it appears that AHCC can actually relieve most and sometimes all of the extremely unpleasant effects of cancer chemotherapy.

Hair Loss Prevention

One of the most psychologically distressing symptoms of chemotherapy is hair loss (alopecia). After doctors began to report that patients taking AHCC were protected against chemotherapy-induced hair loss, medical researchers performed a study on rats. Using an agent to induce hair loss in rats, the researchers showed that the rats using AHCC orally had the most protection from the chemically induced alopecia.

Protects the Bone Marrow

A more dangerous effect of cancer chemotherapy is called *myelosuppression*. Myelosuppression is inhibition of, or damage to bone marrow function. The bone marrow is an important part of the immune system and is the site for red blood cell production. The result of bone marrow damage is low white blood cell counts, which is a cardinal sign of impaired immunity, leaving the patient hypersensitive to infections. Another result is anemia, which contributes to the patient's fatigue and overall loss of resistance. Research in Korea showed that oral treatment with AHCC raised the white blood cell count remarkably in cancer patients who had received chemotherapy. In seven months white blood cell counts averaging below 6,000 were elevated almost to 8,000. Researchers in Japan found that rats were protected from loss of red blood cell production after chemotherapy when protected by the oral use of AHCC.

Prevents Liver Damage

In a Japanese study, rats were given strong chemotherapeutic agents and divided into two groups, one receiving AHCC orally and the other group not. Liver enzyme levels were measured. When there is destruction of liver tissues, there are high levels of the liver enzymes sGOT and sGPT. The group receiving only the chemotherapy agents had large increases in the liver enzymes, but the group that took the drugs with AHCC had normal levels.

Nausea and Vomiting

Nausea and vomiting can be so severe in some cancer patients receiving chemotherapy as to cause them to abandon treatment. The severity of side effects such as this have caused doctors and researchers to measure the benefit of certain kinds of medical treatment against quality of life (QOL). Quality of life surveys have been used as a research tool in recent years to evaluate medical care, particularly in the late stages of illness. Clinical studies in Korea and Japan have indicated that AHCC remarkably improves quality of life, not only in terms of nausea and vomiting, but also in general well-being. All of the three main parameters of QOL were improved by AHCC: physical function and performance, psychological state and social interaction.

AHCC has also been shown to improve appetite in cancer patients undergoing chemotherapy and to help them gain weight. The reduction in psychological stress is of immense benefit to immunity and longevity, as well as general enhancement of life.

AHCC Combined with Chemotherapy

Researchers in Japan analyzed 229 cases of cancer treatment over a three-year period in which 127 were treated with AHCC and the remaining 102 were not. In almost all cases AHCC was used in combination with a conventional chemotherapeutic agent. The mean survival time and mean survival rates were compared with a control group that had not taken AHCC. The results showed that oral treatment with AHCC prolonged the survival times of patients with all types of cancer.

In 1998 a published study showed how AHCC enhanced the therapeutic effects of chemotherapy and reduced the negative effects. AHCC prevented inhibition of NK cell activity by the chemotherapy and enhanced macrophage activity, which is usually suppressed by the drugs. Combined AHCC and conventional chemotherapy enhanced efficiency by decreasing tumor size 20 percent more than the chemotherapy alone and preventing metastasis, spread of cancer to other parts of the body, by 30 percent more than chemotherapy alone. One of the great advantages of AHCC is that conventional chemotherapy does not distinguish between normal cells and cancer cells, but AHCC stimulates the action of the NK (natural killer) cells which destroy only the abnormal cells.

AHCC Combined with Nontoxic Cancer Therapy

One would expect that if AHCC is effective when used along with a toxic chemical used for treating cancer, it would be at least as effective when combined with nontoxic food-derived medications. One substance tested was genistein, a substance derived from soybeans, which is used as an anti-tumor agent. In a study on mice with lung cancer, among four groups—"controls" receiving only water, mice receiving only AHCC, mice receiving only genistein and mice receiving AHCC plus genistein—groups that took AHCC plus genistein lost the most tumor mass after thirty days.

Another therapeutic substance studied with AHCC was an antioxidant derived from buckwheat called *PMP* (polyphenol mixture from plant). Antioxidants are well known for their ability to block cancer at all stages from initiation, promotion and progression. AHCC and PMP had a significant effect in preventing the development of skin cancer in rats.

Another study with breast cancer patients showed that the group treated with AHCC had a higher mean survival rate. At the Comfort Hospital in Yokohama, Japan, AHCC has been used in combination treatment (using a biological response modifier) with over 500 cancer patients with a rate of partial or complete remission in 35 percent of the patients.

AHCC for Hepatitis

Hepatitis is a growing problem in the civilized world. Chronic hepatitis, viral hepatitis type B or C can become liver cancer or liver cirrhosis. Interferon is often used for treatment, but it often does not significantly reduce the viral load and can produce unpleasant side effects such as abdominal pain, anxiety, depression and anemia. AHCC has no side effects and is effective for hepatitis and preventing severe liver degeneration.

We have already seen how AHCC benefits patients by protecting the liver from cytotoxic chemotherapy for cancer both in human clinical trials and in animal studies. In another study, researchers used the toxic chemical carbon tetrachloride with rats to destroy liver cells. Rats given AHCC were protected from the destructive effects of the carbon tetrachloride. In another study, rats were given galactosamine (a substance that can induce acute liver damage) that is fatal in high doses. In a twenty-four-hour period, three of ten mice in the group that took no AHCC died, where all of the mice given AHCC survived. Furthermore, the rats in the AHCC group had significantly lower enzymes, indicating minimal liver destruction.

AHCC has also shown that it can protect the liver from damage resulting from alcohol intake. AHCC can improve swelling of the liver from alcohol consumption and improve serum triglyceride levels. AHCC also prevents liver deterioration in chronic viral hepatitis and low blood platelet count, which can deteriorate into cirrhosis of the liver and liver cancer.

Fred Pescatore, M.D., of Dallas, Texas has reported marked reductions in liver enzymes in hepatitis patients, and has seen the viral loads in hepatitis C patients drop from 200,000 down to 20,000 in as little as two months at a daily dose of 3 grams.

AHCC for Diabetes

Diabetes is one of the most widespread diseases of adults. It is a problem of sugar metabolism caused by lack of insulin, insensitivity to insulin or disordered blood sugar metabolism. Diabetes treatment consists of low glycemic diets, hypoglycemiant (blood sugar-lowering) drugs, exercise, herbs and supplements. Diabetes can have serious complications including frequent infections, muscle cramps, erectile dysfunction, chronic vaginitis, neuritis and other nerve conditions, damage to the eyes, kidneys, heart and peripheral circulation even to the point of lower extremity amputation. The death rate for heart disease and stroke is two to four times higher in diabetics. Several clinicians and researchers have reported that AHCC reduces the blood glucose levels in diabetics.

In a laboratory study with rats, diabetes was induced by injecting a chemical called STZ (streptozotocin) that destroys the insulin-secreting B cells of the Islets of Langerhans in the pancreas. In one group oral AHCC was administered. In the STZ group without AHCC, body weight decreased and even by the second day after STZ administration their general appearance deteriorated. In the group that received STZ plus AHCC, the weight remained steady and the appearance was not affected. Blood glucose levels in the STZ-only group increased, but in the STZ-plus-AHCC group, blood glucose decreased significantly. The STZ-plus-AHCC group showed little damage to the B cells of the Islets of Langerhans compared to the STZ-only group. Insulin levels decreased in the STZ-only group, but increased with the STZ-plus-AHCC group. The results of this study by Amino Up Chemical Company were confirmed by a study at Teikyo University, also in Japan.

A doctor in Japan studied thirteen diabetic patients who were given AHCC over a six-month period. In all of the patients the average blood glucose level, as well as the glycohemoglobin (HbA1c) level, decreased significantly. Blood glucose levels are very changeable and sensitive to external influences, but glycohemoglobin, a combination of glucose (blood sugar) and hemoglobin (the oxygen-carrying component in red blood cells) is a stable indicator of the average glucose level over an extended time period. This is a clear indication of the potential therapeutic effect of AHCC for diabetes.

Cardiovascular Effects of AHCC

AHCC was first developed as a treatment for hypertension. Dr. Fred Pescatore of the Center for Integrative and Complementary Medicine in New York reported that AHCC can prevent stress-induced high blood pressure and damage to the heart. Patients taking AHCC often experience normalization of their blood pressure. Dr. M. Iwamoto of the En-Zan-Kai Medical Corporation reported a beneficial influence of AHCC on ventricular arrhythmias, a type of heart disorder in which the heart rhythm is disrupted.

Effects of AHCC on Stress

A Japanese study at Dokkyo Medical University on rats revealed potential benefits of AHCC for the treatment of stress-related disorders. Under stress the body's production of certain adrenal hormones increases. Stress hormones, such as adrenalin and glucocorticoids (GC) can suppress the responsiveness of the immune system. In the study, rats were subjected to stress from immobilization. Normally, the result of this kind of stress is increased corticosteroid production, increased blood sugar because of high adrenalin secretion and an increase in uric acid levels. When rats were pre-treated with AHCC, they did not show signs of stress and showed no measurable increase in adrenalin, corticosteroid or uric acid levels.

Controlling stress has been recognized in recent years as an important factor in maintaining health. High stress can have deleterious effects on immunity. Stress can be an important factor in heart disease, gastrointestinal disease, nervous system diseases, hormone regulation, pain and many other health problems. AHCC can potentially protect the immune system from many types of disease that could be related to stress.

Effects of AHCC on Infections

The decline in the effectiveness of conventional antibiotics in recent years has been well publicized. Protection from infections in hospitals has become a serious issue for patient safety. Doctors at Teikyo University treated rats with a strong anticancer drug to lower their resistance to infection. The rats were then intravenously inoculated with different microbes to test if AHCC increased their resistance to infection. The microbes used were *Candida albicans*, which causes candidiasis and *Pseudomonas aeruginosa*, which causes pneumonia, some types of ear infections and meningitis. The research showed that AHCC protected the immune system's supply of neutrophils, the white blood cell produced in the bone marrow. It was concluded that the effect of AHCC was to protect the bone marrow cells from damage by the drug.

AHCC has been shown to be effective in protecting patients from opportunistic infections. Opportunistic infections are infections that are apparently caused by suppression of the immune system. Cancer patients are very susceptible to pseudomonas infections. Diabetic patients are also susceptible to pseudomonas and staphylococcus infections. AIDS patients are very susceptible to infections with candida, herpes, pneumocystis and others. According to reports, AHCC gives protection to candida, aspergillus, pseudomonas and a type of *Staphylococcus aureus*, that is especially difficult to control (methicillin-resistant *Staphylococcus aureus*, sometimes called *MRSA*).

The problem of resistance to antibiotics by disease-causing microbes has received a great deal of attention in the media, because it has been a great cause of concern by the medical profession in recent years. Since AHCC helps control infection not by killing pathogenic microbes, but by protecting the immune system's resources. Because of this, there can be no acquired antibiotic resistance to AHCC. AHCC has demonstrated its ability to work synergistically with anticancer drugs. It could be part of the solution to the antibiotic dilemma if it can also work synergistically with the antibiotics that are still effective. The antibiotics themselves weaken the immune system, and AHCC at least can have a protective effect from the negative effects of the antibiotics.

As previously mentioned, doctors and researchers have begun to speculate that the origin of such diseases as cancer. AIDS and other chronic and degenerative diseases is a malfunction of the immune system. Since the late 19th century, microbes have been considered to be the cause of infectious diseases. This point of view is gradually beginning to change. If the cause of infections is poor resistance resulting in high susceptibility, as it appears to be in the case of opportunistic infections, then AHCC can address the original cause of infection by bolstering immunity.

AHCC for Inflammation

Inflammation is a problem not only in infections, but also in acute injuries such as sports injuries and chronic joints and connective tissue problems like arthritis and rheumatism. AHCC has been tested for its efficacy for inflammation both from acute causes as well as chronic disorders. Researchers at Teikyo University found that rats with peritonitis were protected by AHCC taken orally. The results show two things: first, AHCC can improve fat metabolism by raising the levels of the hormone leptin. Second, AHCC modulates the immune system's response.

Control of inflammation is a serious medical problem in that inflammation is often a source of demoralizing chronic pain. Another medical problem of inflammation is the nature of the side effects of treatment. Inflammation is often treated with steroids like cortisone, which do not correct the underlying problem, but only suppress the inflammation and give temporary relief. The terrible side effects of steroids are well known. These side effects can be summarized by saying that steroids suppress the immune system leaving the patient in a state of fatigue and vulnerable to infections. The nonsteroidal anti-inflammatory drugs (often called *NSAIDs*) often have side effects like indigestion, nausea and gastrointestinal bleeding. Some of them also have damaging effects on immunity. The new class of anti-inflammatory drugs, known as Cox-2 inhibitors, seem to have fewer side effects, but they are relatively new and their long-term safety is not known. In any case, anti-inflammatory drugs do not have a corrective effect on the original problem causing the inflammation. AHCC has the potential at least to protect the immune system from the effects of anti-inflammatory drugs, possibly to work with them synergistically, and possibly to improve the underlying cause of the disease.

AHCC and Autoimmune Disease

There is other biochemical evidence of AHCC's beneficial effect on the immune system's ability to control inflammation. Calprotectin, a protein found in neutrophils, increases in the blood serum of patients who have inflammation. Calprotectin destroys the cells it comes in contact with, but AHCC inhibits the destructive effect calprotectin has on cells. In rheumatoid arthritis, calprotectin is found in large amounts in the synovial fluid. This is the lubricating fluid found inside the joints. Dr. Iwamoto of Enzankai Medical Corporation found that a patient taking AHCC to prevent cancer recurrence got relief from his symptoms of rheumatoid arthritis.

The example of rheumatoid arthritis is an important one, because rheumatoid arthritis is an example of an autoimmune disease. Autoimmune diseases are considered by conventional medicine to be diseases in which the immune system attacks cells of the body and causes their destruction. Besides rheumatoid arthritis, SLE (systemic lupus erythematosus), Crohn's disease, multiple sclerosis and numerous other diseases are suspected as being autoimmune. Some conventional as well as alternative medicine doctors are advising not to use substances that stimulate the immune system in the case of autoimmune disease, because the immune system should be suppressed in these cases. It may depend on which type of immunity is being stimulated or suppressed.

If an immune-supporting supplement strengthens humoral immunity, it may offer protection against coughs and colds, but it could possibly at the same time inhibit the cellular immunity. If AHCC can relieve the symptoms of rheumatoid arthritis and slow the progression of the disease, then it may even be used to treat autoimmune diseases by supporting and strengthening the cellular immunity.

Other Health Problems

Clinicians throughout the world have reported benefits from AHCC for health problems that have not actually been the subject of formal scientific studies. Informal studies and anecdotal reports from clinicians point to many possible applications. There has already been considerable cancer research in universities and hospitals. In one informal study in which AHCC was used to treat patients with several different types of cancer, two of three prostate cancer patients had a decline in PSA, prostate specific antigen (a lab index used to diagnose and evaluate prostate cancer), levels. Two of three ovarian cancer patients experienced complete remission. One of three breast cancer patients had a complete remission. One of two multiple myeloma cases experienced complete remission. It is very unusual to see an improvement with this type of cancer. In almost all HIV cases reported, T cell counts can be maintained and even increased. In AIDS, the T cell levels typically drop until they reach dangerously low levels. An increase in T cell counts has been observed in as little as one month along with a significant increase in the activity of NK cells, which are weakened by the presence of HIV. Decreases in intraocular pressure have been reported in cases of glaucoma, as well as reduced blood pressure in hypertensive patients. Improved stamina has been reported in patients with chronic fatigue syndrome. Accelerated healing of slow-healing wounds has been observed. Reduced fat levels in the blood have been seen in patients with hyperlipidemia. Patients have recovered from recurring infections such as colds, influenza, and infections from bacteria, yeast and parasites. Patients have recovered from stomach ulcers, which is also often a bacterial infection from *H. pylori*. Women with a questionable PAP smear, indicating cervical dysplasia or atypia, have taken AHCC with no other form of treatment, and returned to normal, even with PAP readings indicating stage II and stage III dysplasia. Stage II and stage III dysplasia is considered pre-cancerous and is usually treated surgically. The range and variety of afflictions improved by treatment with AHCC continues to grow as more health care practitioners are using it. The limits of its usefulness are not yet established, because it acts on the body's immunity at such a fundamental level.

Who Should Use AHCC?

- People with life-threatening disease
- People with cancer, hepatitis or AIDS should definitely consider what at least is safe immune support, but may even make the difference in survival and longevity
- People with other chronic or degenerative disease
- People with diabetes, heart disease, high blood pressure or autoimmune diseases can benefit by reduction of complications from treatment and possible reversal of the condition
- People with chronic pain
- People with pain from arthritis, injuries, fibromyalgia and anyone regularly using steroids or non-steroidal anti-inflammatory drugs can benefit if not with pain relief, then at least by having fewer damaging side effects of medications
- People with a questionable diagnosis

- Women with cervical dysplasia from diagnosed by a PAP smear, men with an elevated PSA indicating possible prostate problems or anything that can raise fears of a potential dangerous medical condition
- People with a chronic infection
- People infected with candida, staphylococcus, parasitic infestations, herpes or other viral infections can benefit by controlling or eliminating the infection
- People who are exposed to hazardous environmental conditions
- People whose work exposes them to toxic chemicals, and people who expose themselves to lifestyle risks, tobacco, excess alcohol, risky sexual practices, etc.
- People at risk for infectious disease
- People exposed to others during seasonal changes and flu season

Safety and Dosage

AHCC is a completely natural food grade product. It is very safe even at extremely high doses (LD50>12,500 mg/kg). The recommended dose for patients with active cancer is 3 grams daily for two weeks followed by a maintenance dose of a minimum of 1 gram per day. A case of a woman with hepatitis C was reported at the American Academy of Anti-Aging Medicine in which she took 6 grams of AHCC per day. Her viral load decreased 89 percent in four months and was normal after seven months. It is possible that higher doses are more beneficial. Doses of 6 grams per day have also been used for immune protection in patients undergoing chemotherapy for cancer.

Cost may discourage some people from experimenting with very high doses, but the cost-effectiveness of AHCC compares favorably with many immune stimulants, particularly when one considers its versatility, safety and reliability. Therapy with the cytokine IL-2 (interleukin-2) can cost as much as $100,000. Interferon treatment can be expensive and unpleasant. AHCC increases the body's own production of IL-2 and interferon without having to resort to an expensive outside source.

How to Use AHCC

For any type of chronic problem, it would be advisable to start out with a loading dose of 3 grams per day for one to two weeks, depending on the severity and chronic nature of the problem. There is often measurable improvement after two weeks. For life-threatening disease, the dose of 3 grams per day should be maintained for at least three months. How soon one can expect symptomatic relief depends on the nature of the problem as well. In all cases it is advisable to seek the advice of a health care professional.

People taking prescription drugs should inform the prescribing physician and seek cooperation in evaluating the effects of AHCC in case of possible synergistic effects. No negative side effects or drug interactions with AHCC have been reported during the history of its use. On the contrary, AHCC has been reported to relieve unpleasant side effects of drugs, even toxic, dangerous cancer chemotherapy drugs.

References

Abe S, Ishibashi H, Inoue Y, Tansho S, Ikeda T, Ono Y, Yamaguchi H, "Preventive effect of AHCC on opportunistic infection and its mechanism," AHCC Research Association 8th Symposium, Sapporo, Japan, 2000.

Ahn GH, Han US, "Prospective, randomized, clinical evaluation of QOL & immune index of AHCC in advanced metastatic cancer patients," AHCC Research Association 8th Symposium, Sapporo, Japan, 2000.

Buttyan R, Katx A, Cao Y, Dorai T, Olsson C, "A mixture of basidiomycetes polysaccharides and genistein (GCP) inhibits proliferation and induces apoptosis in human prostate cancer cells in vitro and in vivo," AHCC Research Association 8th Symposium, Sapporo, Japan, 2000.

Ghoneum M, "NK-immunomodulation by active hemicellulose compound in 17 cancer patients," *Society of Natural Immunity*, Taormina, Italy May 25-28, 1994, p.56.

Ghoneum M, et al, "Enhancement of human NK cell activity in vivo by active hemicellulose compound (AHCC)," Abstract of the 7th Annual Conference on Clinical Immunology, November 13-15, 1992.

Ghoneum M, Ninomiya Y, Torabi M, Gill G, Wojdani A, "Active hemicellulose compound enhances NK cell activity of aged mice in vivo," Abstract of Federation Association Society of Experimental Biology Meeting, April 5-9, 1992.

Ghoneum M, Wimbley M, Salem F, McKlain A, Attalah N, Gill G, "Immunomodulatory and anti-cancer effects of active hemicellulose compound (AHCC)," *International Journal of Immunotherapy* XI (1) 23-28 (1995)

Ginaldi L, De Martinis M, d'Ostilio A, Marini L, Loreto MF, Corsi MP, "The immune system in the elderly: I. Specific Humoral Immunity," *Immunol Res* 1999; 20(2):101-108.

Hagiwara M, Yanagawa C, "Experience of AHCC on progressive, residual and recurrent cancer - Preliminary report," AHCC Research Association 8th Symposium, Sapporo, Japan, 2000.

Hosokawa M, Matsushita K, "Combination of AHCC and chemotherapy," AHCC Research Association 8th Symposium, Sapporo, Japan, 2000.

Ishiguro A, et al, "Anti-carcinogenic activity of AHCC and PMP," The 2nd Annual Meeting of the Japanese Society of Alternative Medicine and Treatment, Oct 1999.

Ishizaki M, Matsui Y, Kawaguchi Y, Kamiyama Y, "Case report: Inhibition of liver cirrhosis progression in a case of C type hepatitis with hepatocellular carcinoma," AHCC Research Association 8th Symposium, Sapporo, Japan, 2000.

Iwamoto M, "A clinical study for AHCC on chronic hepatitis patients," AHCC Research Association 8th Symposium, Sapporo, Japan, 2000.

Iwamoto M, et al, "A study on dose-dependence of AHCC for cancer patients," The 2nd Annual Meeting of the Japanese Society of Alternative Medicine and Treatment, Oct 1999.

Iwamoto M, et al, "Effects of AHCC on diabetes from clinical and basic research," The 2nd Annual Meeting of the Japanese Society of Alternative Medicine and Treatment, Oct 1999.

Kanazawa T, et al, "The components in AHCC activating macrophages and inhibiting tumor cell proliferation," The 5th Research Association of Cancer Prevention, July, 1998.

Kawaguchi Y, Teshima S, Toyokawa H, Sugimoto N, Matsumiya M, Araki H, Komada N, Kamiyama Y, "Effect of AHCC on digestive cancer—especially for terminal cancer," AHCC Research Association 8th Symposium, Sapporo, Japan, 2000.

Kosuna K, "The Development and Application of Active Hemocellulose Compound) (AHCC)," *Bio Industry* September 1993, Volume 10.

Kosuna K, "Recent Progress of Research on AHCC; Active Hexose Correlated Compound," *New Food Industry*, 41, 17-23, 2000.

Matsui Y, Ishizaki M, Kitade H, Morita H, Kawaguchi Y, Kamiyama Y, "Effects of AHCC as a complementary treatment for postoperative hepatocellular carcinoma patients," AHCC Research Association 8th Symposium, Sapporo, Japan, 2000.

Matsui Y, Kawaguchi Y, Nakagawa M, Hon-Kwon A, Kamiyama Y, Kosuna K, "Preventive effects of active hexose correlated compound (AHCC) on the recurrence of postoperative hepatocellular carcinoma patients," XXXIIIrd Congress of the European Society for Surgical Research, 1998, p.74.

Matsushita K, Kuramitsu Y, Ohiro Y, Obara M, Kobayashi M, Li YQ, Hosokawa M, "Combination therapy of active hexose correlated compound plus UFT significantly reduces the metastasis of rat mammary adenocarcinoma," *Anti-Cancer Drugs* 1998, Vol. 9, pp.343-350.

Matsuzaki S, Wang S, Ichimura K, Wakame K, Kosuna K, "Preventive effect of AHCC on oxidative stress," AHCC Research Association 8th Symposium, Sapporo, Japan, 2000.

Mukoda T, Sun B, Kosuna K, "Active hexose correlated compound (AHCC) protects against cytosine arabinoside induced alopecia in the newborn rat animal model," *Japanese Journal of Cancer Research* 1989, 2405.

Pescatore F, "Role of AHCC as a part of an adult disease treatment protocol," AHCC Research Association 8th Symposium, Sapporo, Japan, 2000.

Sun B, "Improving effect of active hexose correlated compound (AHCC) on liver injury induced by anti-cancer drugs," The 119th Meeting of the Japanese Society of Pharmacology, Mar 1999.

Sun B, et al, "Anti-carcinogenic effect of AHCC and buckwheat polyphenol," The 37th Meeting of the Japanese Society of Cancer Treatment, Oct 1999.

Sun B, et al, "Anti-mutagenic effects of AHCC," The 4th Research Association of Cancer Prevention, May, 1997.

Sun B, et al, "Fractions of AHCC (active hexose correlated compound) and their effects on macrophages and tumor cell lines," The 57th Annual Meeting of the Japanese Cancer Association, Sep 1998.

Sun B, Fukuhara M, Kosuna K, "Reduction of side effects of anti-cancer drugs by AHCC, mycelial extracts of cultures basidiomycetes," Impact of Biotechnology on Cancer, Nice, France, Nov 1998.

Sun B, Kosuna K, "Effects of AHCC (active hexose correlated compound) in both the prevention and treatment of carcinoma," Critical Appraisal of

Inconventional/Alternative Interventions for Carcinoma of the Prostate, May, 1998.

Sun B, Shi X, White R, Hackman R, "Various effects of the co-administration of AHCC and GCP (genistein concentrated polysaccharide) in vitro and in vivo." AHCC Research Association 8th Symposium, Sapporo, Japan, 2000.

Sun B, Wakame K, Mukota T, Toyoshima A, Kanazawa T, Kosuna K, "Protective effects of AHCC on carbon tetrachloride-induced liver injury in mice," *Natural Medicine*, 51, 310-315, 1997.

Tasaki S, Kamiyama Y, et al, "Immunotherapy with AHCC in hepatocellular carcinoma epatients," The 32nd Congress of the European Society for Surgical Research, May 1997.

Uno K, Chikumaru S, Hosokawa T, "Cancer immunotherapy by a phyto-poly-saccharide (AHCC): its effects and strategy," AHCC Research Association 8th Symposium, Sapporo, Japan, 2000.

Uno K, et al, "Active hexose correlated compound (AHCC) improves immunological parameters and performance status of patients with solid tumors," *Biotherapy*, 14(3): 303-307, May 2000.

Wakame K, "Protective effects of active hexose correlated compound (AHCC) on the onset of diabetes induced by streptozotocin in the rat," *Biomedical Research* 20 (3) 145-152, 1999.

Yui S, Yamazaki M, "Regulatory effect of AHCC on inflammation," AHCC Research Association 8th Symposium, Sapporo, Japan, 2000.

About the Author

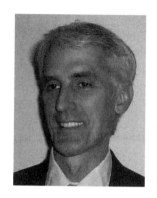

Dan Kenner is licensed to practice oriental medicine in Japan and the U.S. He has a Ph.D. in naturopathic medicine and has studied European naturopathic approaches to medicine, including German biological medicine and French phytoaromatherapy. He is the author of *Botanical Medicine: A European Professional Perspective* (Paradigm, 1996). Dr. Kenner is on the board of directors of Meiji College of Oriental Medicine and the California Institute of Integrative Medicine in Santa Rosa, California and teaches at the First National University of Naturopathic Medicine and various other educational institutions in the U.S., Europe and east Asia.

Woodland Health Series

Definitive Natural Health Information At Your Fingertips!

The Woodland Health Series offers a comprehensive array of single topic booklets, covering subjects from fibromyalgia to green tea to acupressure. If you enjoyed this title, look for other WHS titles at your local health-food store, or contact us. Complete and mail (or fax) us the coupon below and receive the complete Woodland catalog and order form—free!

Or . . .

- Call us toll-free at **(800) 777-2665**
- Visit our website (**www.woodlandpublishing.com**)
- Fax the coupon (and other correspondence) to **(801) 785-8511**

Woodland Publishing Customer Service

P.O. BOX 160 • PLEASANT GROVE, UTAH • 84062

❑ *YES! Send me a free Woodland Publishing catalog.*
❑ *YES! Send me a free issue of the* WOODLAND HEALTH REPORT *newsletter.*

Name _____

Address _____

_____

_____

City _____ State _____ Zip Code _____

Phone _____ email _____